The Jerk Journal

Let It All Out

CATIE HARRIS

IWJTPodcast.com/Catie Harris

ISBN-13: 978-0-9982519-8-1

Dedicated to:
My son, my true inspiration
Matthew Harris

A lot of people have a lot of opinions of how to deal with jerks in the workplace. But no resolution comes close to the catharsis of just saying what you think.

Of course saying what you think isn't without consequences. I said what I thought of my attending to his face and got suspended for 2 days. No one defended me, came to my rescue or thanked me for standing up to the jerk. Instead, I got suspended without pay for 2 days, lessons in anger management for several weeks and a "record" of bad behavior in Human Resources.

The irony of my situation is that it came about because I had kept my mouth shut for so long. In general I don't want to make mountains out of molehills, or bother other people or feel like I couldn't just "handle it".

Ultimately though all the negative energy simmered inside me and boiled over in a crazy, ranting session. It was a catharsis that occurred.

Neither situation is ideal. You can't and maybe shouldn't always confront the jerk, especially when he or she controls your paycheck, and you can't keep it inside. Trust me, the anger will eat you alive!

What's the alternative?

Now let's be clear. I'm not telling you what to do or that you should do this, but here is what I do. I also did not make this tidbit up, I stole the idea from Abraham Lincoln. Abraham Lincoln is quite possibly one of the most diplomatic and successful negotiators that we know about. He always spoke well of others and even went to great lengths to be friendly to his enemies.

Why? Because it was effective. Didn't he hate his enemies? Of course, he was human after all! Here is the trick he did to control his reaction outwardly.

Abe used to write letters to the people he hated. He would say exactly what he wanted in the way he wanted to. He would get all his emotions out and tell off the SOB at the other end of his letter. And then he could sleep. He felt emotionally spent and exhausted. The letter would go inside his desk and never leave his clutches.

The great thing is that Abe never hung on to anger. He always said exactly how he felt, and the result was the same.

Abe didn't have to suffer the consequences of saying things he could never take back, but he reaped all the rewards of saying things he wanted to in a letter.

I've used this tactic in the past for jerky co-workers, jerky ex-boyfriends, and just plain jerks. It is amazing how powerful writing your thoughts out can be!

Again this is not novel, the American Psychological Association endorses research that shows that writing can strengthen the immune system, improve well-being and provide a litany of health benefits.

Now look, there will be times when you need to confront others, talk about situations and employ other mechanisms depending on your situation, but writing out your thoughts first is an excellent way to experience a massive catharsis.

Don't let a jerk cause poor health in your life. The worst revenge you can have is to lead a happy, healthy and prosperous life! So get ready to unleash all in your very own Jerk Journal. Always remember to keep it somewhere that no one will find it!

And get started. Right. Now.

Catie

Dear ______________________

Dear ________________________

Dear ______________________

Dear ________________________

Dear ____________________

Dear ____________________

Dear ______________________

Dear ________________________

Dear ______________________

Dear ____________________

Dear ____________________

Dear ________________________

Dear ____________________

Dear ______________________

Dear ____________________

Dear ____________________

Dear ______________________

Dear ______________________________

Dear

Dear ________________________

Dear ____________________

Dear ________________________

Dear ___________________

Dear ____________________

Dear ________________________________

Dear ______________________

Dear ____________________

Dear ____________________

Dear ____________________

Dear ____________________

Dear

Dear ______________________

Dear ___________________

Dear ______________________

Dear ____________________

Dear ______________________

Dear ______________________

Dear ________________________

Dear ______________________

Dear ______________________________

Dear ______________________

Dear ______________________________

Dear ______________________

Dear ____________________

Dear

Dear ______________________

Dear ____________________

Made in the USA
Monee, IL
06 May 2026

49633083R00109